COCONUT OIL MIRACLE HANDBOOK

A Simple Guide on the health benefits and uses of Coconut Oil

By

Dr. Tee Stevens

Contents

PREFACE

This book on Coconut oil will particularly teach you on the benefits and health benefits of the coconut oil. The book will simply guide you on what coconut oil entails, types of coconut oil, health benefits of coconut oil, coconut oil recipes and so many more.

INTRODUCTION

Coconut oil is a kind of tropical oil derived from the nut or meat of the coconut palm. Sold as an oil or added to cosmetic products, candles, and prepared foods; the coconut oil comprises of medium-chain fatty acids, such as caprylic acid, lauric acid, as well as capric acid.

Coconut oil has a humidifying effect when applied to the skin and around 52% to 85% of coconut oil comprises of specific **_saturated fats,_** referred to as medium-chain fatty acids.

Coconut oil is commonly used by individuals for the treatment of eczema as well as growth in premature infants. Nevertheless, it is also used for condition such as obesity, breast cancer, heart disease, psoriasis, as well as multiple sclerosis, although there is no significant scientific proof to ascertain these uses as numerous experts have questioned just how healthy it is.

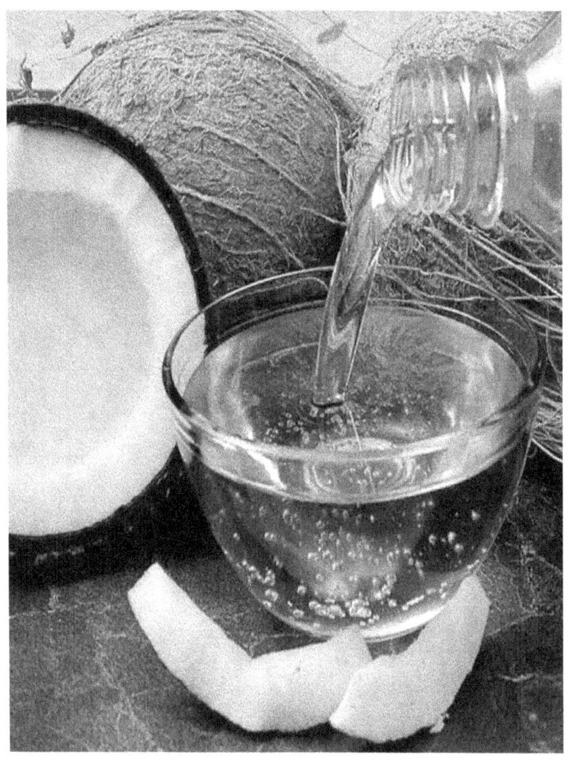

Coconut oil which is usually promoted as a keto-friendly food enjoyed a burst of popularity that has waned currently.

Nutritional component of one (1) tablespoon serving of coconut oil comprises of

Protein	0 grams
Fiber	0 grams
Sugar	0 grams
Saturated Fat	11.2 grams
Calories	121
Carbohydrates	0 grams
Fat	11.5 grams
Choline	0.04 mg
Vitamin K	0.082 mcg
Vitamin E	0.015 mg
Calcium	0.14 mg
Monounsaturated fat	0.86 grams
Polyunsaturated Fat	0.23 grams

Despite the fact that coconut oil possesses a similar nutritional component to other cooking oils, the primary difference lies in the exact type of fat it contains. The majority (83%) of the fat in coconut oil is saturated fat and this is the kind of fat generally found in animal products such as dairy and meat. On the flip side, only about 14% of the fat is **saturated** in olive oil.

At room temperature, saturated fat tends to be solid and usually considered unhealthy since there is proof that diets high in saturated fats increase LDL (low density lipoprotein) or *"bad"* cholesterol levels, which in turn raise the risk of heart disease. Contrarily, unsaturated fats, either monounsaturated or polyunsaturated, stay liquid at room temperature and are preconceived healthier because in moderation, and particularly in place of saturated fats, they have been demonstrated to have a useful effect on the health of the heart.

A single tablespoon (tbsp) of coconut oil closely follows the American Heart Association's recommended 13g per day limit on saturated fat (in relation to a 2,000-calorie-per-day diet).

Concurrently, the same amount of olive comprises of less than 2 g of saturated fat and for that particular reason, numerous experts assert that olive is a healthier option. As a result of its saturated fat content, coconut oil has acquired a recognition as an unhealthy, artery-clogging oil and numerous experts still suggest avoiding the coconut oil. However, in current years, some researchers have questioned whether saturated fat is as unhealthy as initially speculated, and there is been renewed interest in coconut oil as a potential healthy choice.

Coconut Oil and its dosage

There is literally no standard recommended dosage of coconut oil, although less than or equal to one tablespoon of coconut oil each day is recommended based on the following regulations:

(a) The present dietary guidelines for Americans suggest consuming no more than 10% of total calories from saturated fat. Based on a 2,000 calorie diet, this is equal to 200 calories and around 22 grams of saturated fat which is equal to less than 2 tablespoons (tbsp) of coconut oil. It also entails that you would be required to reduce all other sources of saturated fat in your diet, such as full-fat dairy products as well as animal fat.

(b) One tablespoon of coconut oil comprises of 13.5 grams of saturated fat.

(c) For individuals at risk of who already have a heart disease, the American Heart Association recommends no more than 6% of total calories from saturated fat,

or around 13 grams of saturated
fat from all sources.

CHAPTER ONE

TYPES OF COCONUT OIL

Coconut oil comes in different forms and some products carry several labels.

1. **Unrefined Coconut Oil-** The Unrefined coconut oil directly comes from the meat or nut of the coconut palm. Least processed and unfiltered choice, the unrefined coconut oil does not go through any processing to make the ultimate product more hydrogenated, which is a means to convert unsaturated fatty acids into saturated fatty acids.

   The unrefined coconut oil can be used in recipes in which you want to have a strong coconut taste since it has a more pungent coconut smell and flavor. The unrefined coconut oil has a smoke point of about 350°F, the temperature to which it can be heated before it begins to smoke and demean.

In contrary to olive oil, the terminologies *"virgin" and "extravirgin"* are not regulated with coconut oil as there is no disparity in products labeled with these terms.

2. **Organic Coconut Oil-** Organic coconut oil implies that the coconuts from which the oil has been derived were cultivated in conformity with the requirements of organic agriculture and this refers to the use of herbicides and pesticides, additives, soil quality, among other components.

3. **Refined Coconut Oil-** The refined coconut oil is often derived from dried coconut meat and further

processed to make it better for cooking. After refined coconut oil is pressed from the coconut, it may pass through a few extra steps. Refined coconut oil may be mixed with a degumming agent to eliminate gums (impurities) and then may be neutralized with sodium hydroxide, which acts like soap when mixed with the present fatty acids. The free fatty acids are eliminated during this process, which aids in decreasing the risk of refined coconut oil becoming sour.

Making use of an activated clay filter, refined coconut oil may also be bleached to make it whiter and more uniform and then deodorized to make it tasteless and odorless. Oftentimes, chemical solvents such as *hexane* may be used in extracting oil from the dried coconut meat and after all this processing, refined coconut acquires a higher smoke point of about 400°F to 500°F thus allowing it more culinary versatility than unrefined coconut oil.

CHAPTER TWO

BENEFITS AND HEALTH BENEFITS OF COCONUT OIL

Coconut oil is used in several ways, from cooking to personal care, although individuals may tend to wonder if it is healthy and while there are numerous personal accounts of its benefits, coconut oil lacks sufficient scientific evidence to ascertain these claims.

A lack of research does not automatically imply that coconut oil is not beneficial, although it is helpful to examine study findings when making an evaluation of its benefits.

Coconut oil is a rising popular cooking oil with many individuals praising the oil for its health benefits, such as antioxidant properties, enhanced skin, oral health as well as weight loss potential.

Coconut oil is beneficial in decreasing hunger, improving oral health, decreasing seizures, increasing good cholesterol, controlling blood sugar, decreasing stress, fighting candida albicans, preventing liver disease, decreasing asthma symptoms, and much more.

Numerous products such as *fried foods, shampoos, coffee, smoothies, as well as sweets* comprise of coconut oil.

In 2016, results of a survey in United States of America demonstrated that 72% of individuals believed that coconut oil was healthful, although only 37% of nutritionists agreed.

Coconut oil comprises of over 80% saturated fat with some experts having linked saturated fats with cardiovascular and other disease conditions.

Dietary Guidelines for Americans (2015 to 2020) recommend reducing consumption of saturated fats to less than 10% of day's calories and this entails that an individual following a 2000 calorie per day diet should consume no more than 20g of saturated fat per day.

Some of the benefits and health benefits of coconut oil include:

1. **May work as an instant source of energy-** The medium chain triglycerides (MCTs) in coconut oil offers an instant supply of energy and when you consume *long chain triglycerides,* they are packaged into molecules referred to as ***Chylomicrons*** that are transported into your blood through the lymphatic system. As soon as chylomicrons leave your lymphatic system, they are

moved to your liver and other tissues where they are stored or broken down for energy. Thus, obtaining energy from *long chain triglycerides* take some time.

Conversely, medium chain triglycerides are absorbed intact from the small intestine into the blood and can be quickly used for energy, in much the same manner as carbs- your body's approved source of energy. And as a matter of fact, *medium chain triglycerides* have been long used in sports nutrition products for athletes who require a source of energy their body can absorb and use instantly.

2. **May promote fat burning-** Coconut oil is an excellent source of *medium chain triglycerides,* a kind of saturated fat that get absorbed and metabolized

instantly into the body. *Medium chain triglycerides* can help individuals to feel full, burn extra calories and prevent the bodies from storing the oil as fat. Researchers are studying medium chain triglycerides, including those found in coconut oil, for their potential health uses and benefits.

A 2023 study found that medium-chain triglyceride supplementation, when used during a low-calorie ketogenic diet, remarkably reduced body weight, waist circumference and body mass index. Considering that the fats in coconut oil are 65% medium-chain triglyceride, it may contain fat-burning properties that are like pure *medium-chain triglyceride oil.* It is also vital to keep in mind that coconut oil is extremely rich in calories and can easily result into weight gain if you eat it in large quantities.

3. **May help decrease hunger-** One fascinating characteristic or feature of *medium chain triglycerides* is that they may increase satiety (feeling of fullness) and help decrease intake of food. This may be connected to how the body breaks them down. A segment of medium chain triglycerides you consume are broken down in a process that give rise to molecules known as **ketones.**

   Ketones decrease appetite by either directly acting on the brain's chemical messengers or modifying the levels of hunger-inducing hormones like **ghrelin.**

Nevertheless, although coconut oil is one of the richest sources of *medium chain triglycerides,* there is no proof that coconut oil itself decreases appetite more than oils and as a matter of fact, a study in 2017 reports that coconut oil is less filling than *medium chain triglyceride oil.*

4. **May Enhance the health of Skin-** Coconut oil has numerous uses that have little to do with eating with numerous individuals using it for cosmetic purposes to boost their health and appearance of their skin.

    Studies demonstrate that coconut oil can improve the moisture content of dry skin. It may also boost the function of the skin, helping avoid excessive loss of water as well as protecting you from external factors like chemical, allergens and infectious agents.

As a matter of fact, a study in 2021 ascertained that applying about 6 to 8 drops of virgin coconut oil on your hands and leaving it all through the night may be an efficient way of preventing dry skin caused by regular use of alcohol-based hand sanitizers.

The use of coconut oil may also decrease the severity of mild to moderate symptoms of **atopic dermatitis,** a chronic skin disease depicted by skin inflammation and distortions in skin barrier function. Coconut oil when applied to the skin of premature infants might boost body temperature, skin health, breathing and general growth.

5. **May contain antimicrobial properties-** Coconut oil contains antimicrobial and antifungal properties as a result of its *medium chain triglyceride* content- particularly, *lauric acid.*

Lauric acid is a fatty acid that constitutes around 50% of the *medium chain triglycerides* in coconut oil.

Research indicates that coconut oil may have antimicrobial properties against disease-causing microorganisms, *such as Helicobacter pylori, Escherichia coli, Streptococcus mutans, Streptococcus pyogenes and Staphylococcus aureus.*

Studies demonstrate that lauric acid may act as a bacteriostatic agent and this is a substance that prevents bacteria from multiplying without destroying the bacteria. Furthermore, it may also act as a bacteriocidal agent which kills some bacteria as well as may also inhibit the growth of microorganisms that are toxic to plants.

It has been reported that lauric acid increase HDL cholesterol, protecting the heart and thus take longer time to absorb and metabolize.

6. **May help decrease seizure-** Individuals have long used keto diets, which are extremely low in carbs and rich in fats, to treat several disorders, such as drug-resistant epilepsy in children and they have demonstrated to help decrease how often seizures occur.

It is believed that the lack of available glucose to fuel brain cells is a probable explanation for the decrease in seizure frequency in individuals with epilepsy on ketogenic diets.

Nevertheless, generally, there is a lack of evidence for the use of keto diets in adults with epilepsy and thus more research is required.

Decreasing your intake of carb decreases the glucose in the blood, and increasing your intake of fat leads to remarkably increased concentrations of ketones. Your brain can make use of ketones as a source of energy rather than glucose.

It is demonstrated that the *medium chain triglycerides* in coconut oil get transported to the liver and thus turns into ketones.

7. **May Boost oral health-** A study in 2020 found that making use of

coconut oil as a mouthwash (oil pulling) benefit oral hygiene economically.

Oil pulling involves whizzing coconut oil in your mouth like mouthwash as it may remarkably decrease the count of toxic bacteria in the mouth namely *Streptococcus mutans* as compared with a frequent mouthwash.

This is believed to be as a result of the antibacterial properties of lauric acid.

Furthermore, lauric acid in coconut oil reacts with saliva to form a soap-like substance that fends off cavities and helps in decreasing dental plaque accumulation and gum inflammation.

Nevertheless, studies also demonstrate that oil pulling does not replace dental therapy and thus additional research is required.

8. **May protect against hair damage-** Coconut oil act as a form of protection against hair damage.

   A study in 2021 ascertained that, since coconut oil deeply penetrates hair strands, it makes them more flexible and increases their durability to avert them from breaking under tension.

   In a similar fashion, another study ascertained that coconut oil nourishes hair strands and decreases breakage, which further strengthens the hair.

9. **May act as an excellent source of antioxidant-** Coconut oil is an excellent source of antioxidants, which may help in neutralizing damaging molecules known as

free molecules. This, in turn, helps decrease the risk of various chronic and degenerative diseases.

Polyphenols, flavonoids, tocotrienols, tocopherols, and phytosterols are some of the major types of antioxidants in coconut oil.

10. **May help in decreasing symptoms of Alzheimer's disease-** One of the most common cause of dementia is Alzheimer's disease with the condition decreasing your brain's ability to use glucose for energy. Nevertheless, it is believed that ketones can offset initial or early signs of mild to moderate Alzheimer's disease by providing a different energy source for brain cells.

As a result of this, individual foods such as coconut oil have been examined for their potential role in managing or treating Alzheimer's disease. Nevertheless, additional studies in humans are required.

11. **May help to reduce symptoms of Eczema-** Coconut oil when applied to the skin can decrease symptoms of eczema in children more than applying mineral oil.

CHAPTER THREE

COCONUT OIL RECIPES

At room temperature, coconut oil remains solid but stable at high temperature as a result of its saturated fatty acids. This makes it appropriate for numerous things such as mixing into dressings or sauces, making homemade soups or stews or sautéing eggs or vegetables.

Melted coconut oil can be used rather than any other cooking oil in baking like cookies, cakes and bars. To prevent clumped batter, make sure any eggs and milk you are making use of are at room temperature before blending in the coconut oil. Coconut oil can be enjoyed by adding 1 to 2 teaspoons to drinks like juice, smoothies, tea, and coffee.

Coconut oil is a natural moisturizer which is excellent for your hands, legs, cuticles, and other parts of the body. Coconut oil has been found to boost skin disorders such as eczema and dermatitis and again, it can repair chapped lips and cracked heels.

Coconut oil decreases protein loss from hair when it was applied before or after shampoo and this is as a result of the lauric acid excellent structure that penetrates the hair shaft.

Advantages of cooking with coconut oil

(a) Readily available and less costly than numerous other alternative oils.

(b) Increases good cholesterol and maintains healthy fats when heated, as it withstands higher temperatures than other oils.

(c) Excellent taste and texture, particularly organic extra-virgin coconut oil.

(d) Vegan-diet and dairy free friendly.

(e) Versatile for numerous uses- from baking cakes to frying veggies.

Disadvantages of cooking with coconut oil

(a) When compared to alternative oil such as olive oil or butter, coconut oil is high in calories.

(b) Coconut oil may cause carcinogens to release after continuous deep-frying due to its low smoking point (339.8°F) and thus not suitable for deep frying.

(c) Coconut oil is high in saturated fats thus accounting for 13g of an individual day to day intake.

COCONUT OIL RECIPES

Coconut oil	Requirements	Cooking directions

recipes		
Chocolate chip cookies with coconut oil	2 eggs ¾ cup liquid-form coconut oil ¾ cup white sugar ¾ cup packed brown sugar 2½ cups flour ¾ teaspoon salt 1 cup chocolate chips 2 teaspoons vanilla extract	(a) Preheat oven to 375°F and whisk together liquid coconut oil, eggs, vanilla, and both sugars in a big mixing bowl. (b) Stir in flour, baking soda, and salt until ingredients are mixed and the

| | | dough is smooth and then fold in chocolate chips until they are evenly distributed. |
| | | (c) Line a big baking sheet with parchment paper and scoop dough about 1 inch apart and then |

		bake for around 9 t0 12 minutes or until lightly browne d. (d) Place or put on wire rack to cool.
Apple Cinnam on Granola	¾ cup coconut oil, melted. ½ cup honey. 2 tablespoons pure maple syrup. 1 tablespoon apple pie spice. 1 cup dried	(a) Preheat oven to 250°F and line a sheet pan with parchme nt paper. (b) Spray with non- stick cooking

	apple chips. ½ teaspoon cinnamon. ½ teaspoon kosher salt. ½ cup pecans, chopped. 4 cups old-fashioned rolled oats. ½ cup light brown sugar. ¾ cups chopped walnuts.	spray and whisk together the brown sugar, maple syrup, coconut oil, apple sauce, apple pie spice, cinnamon, and salt in a small bowl. (c) Stir in the oats with the pecans and walnuts

		in a medium-sized bowl and pour the wet mixture over the dry and stir properly to coat and mix all ingredients. (d) Transfer the wet granola to a big baking sheet in a thin and even layer

		and bake for about 1 hour or until golden brown and toasted, stirring once halfway through. (e) Discard from oven for around 15 to 20 minutes and avoid stirring. (f) Add apple chips and blend.

| Roast Carrot Coconut Soup | 2 tablespoons olive oil. 1 tablespoon chopped fresh ginger and coconut oil. 2 pounds carrots, peeled and chopped into one (1) inch pieces. 1 onion. 4 garlic cloves. 3 cups vegetable stock. 1 lime, juiced. Pepper and kosher salt. 2 scallions, thinly | (a) Preheat oven to 425°F and place carrots on a baking sheet and toss with the olive oil. (b) Sprinkle with pepper and salt and then roast for around 20 to 25 minutes or until golden. (c) Heat coconut oil in a |

	sliced. One 14-oz can coconut milk.	pot and as soon as it is melted, stir in onions, ginger, garlic and little salt and pepper. (d) Cook, stirring constant ly, until softens for around 5 to 6 minutes and as soon as carrots are ready, add to the pot

		along with the stock. (e) Bring mixture to a bowl and then decrease to a simmer and cook for around 10 minutes. (f) Gently transfer the mixture to a blender and blend until pureed

		and then pour the soup back into the pot and heat on low.
		(g) Stir in coconut milk and lime juice until the soup is warmed and then season with extra salt and pepper as required.

		(h) Serve with a drizzle of coconut milk and scallions (sliced) on top.
Roast Brussels Sprouts	1 pound Brussels sprouts, trimmed and washed. 2 tablespoons of melted coconut oil. Salt and pepper. 3 tablespoons balsamic vinegar.	(a) Preheat oven to 375°F and slice Brussels sprouts in half and place in a big bowl. (b) Pour balsamic vinegar over the halves, toss to coat and

		add melted coconut oil and then toss again. (c) Into a single layer on a baking sheet, arrange Brussels and sprinkle with pepper and salt. (d) Roast for around 25 minutes or when lightly golden,

		turning the pan after about 10 minutes.
Coconut Oil Apple Muffins	1 cup grated apple. 1 ¾ cups white or whole wheat flour. 2 eggs at room temp. 1 teaspoon ground cinnamon. ½ teaspoon salt. 1/3 cup melted coconut oil. 1 cup apple diced into ¼ cubes.	(a) Preheat oven to 425°F and grease muffin cups with butter or non-stick cooking spray. (b) Whisk together flour, baking soda, baking powder, cinnamo

½ cup maple syrup. ½ cup applesauce. 1 teaspoon vanilla extract. ½ cup plain greek yogurt. ½ teaspoon baking soda and 1 ½ teaspoons baking powder.	n, and salt in a big mixing bowl. (c) Stir in the diced and grated apple and beat the oil and honey/ maple syrup with a whisk in a medium mixing bowl. (d) Then, beat in eggs, accomp

		ained by the applesauce, vanilla,and yogurt, and blend thoroughly. (e) Pour wet ingredients into dry ones and blend until just combined and then divide the batter uniformly

| | | between 12 muffin cups and sprinkle tops with raw sugar. |
| | | (f) Bake for around 13 to 16 minutes, or until golden on top and a toothpick inserted in the middle comes out clean and then place on |

		a cooling rack prior to serving.

Coconut oil is a kind of tropical oil derived from the nut or meat of the coconut palm. Sold as an oil or added to cosmetic products, candles, and prepared foods; the coconut oil comprises of medium-chain fatty acids, such as *caprylic acid, lauric acid, as well as capric acid.*

Coconut oil has a humidifying effect when applied to the skin and around 52% to 85% of coconut oil comprises of specific **saturated fats,** referred to as medium-chain fatty acids.

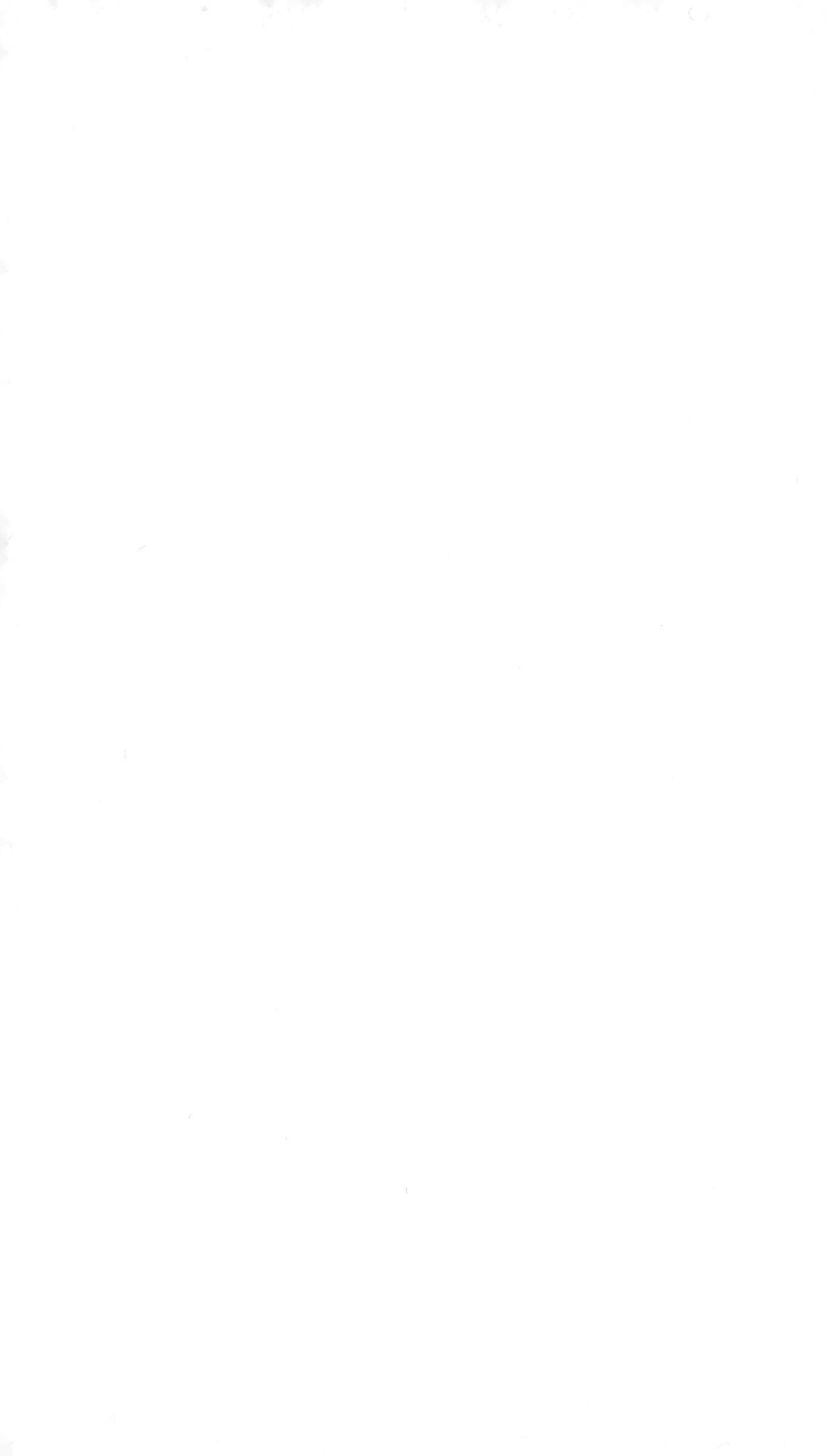

www.ingramcontent.com/pod-product-compliance
Lightning Source LLC
Chambersburg PA
CBHW051709250726
48653CB00007B/2943